P9-EAO-428

# The Master Cleanser

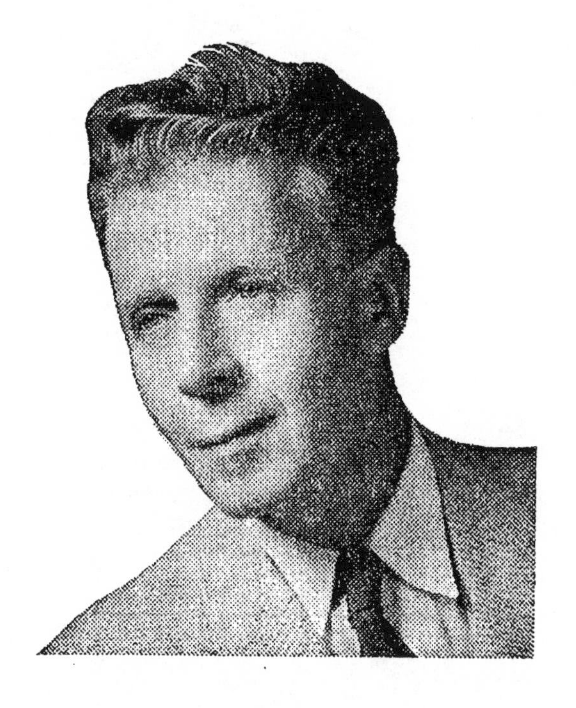

By

Stanley A. Burroughs

3859 Mt. Rubidoux Drive — Riverside, California

**www.snowballpublishing.com**

**info@snowballpublishing.com**

For information regarding special discounts for bulk purchases, please contact Snowball Publishing at

sales@snowballpublishing.com

*"Let no man refuse to listen and be healed lest he bring suffering to those who look to him for guidance.."*

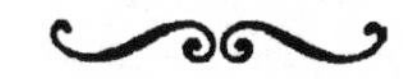

# THE MASTER CLEANSER

Man's mastery of disease will only be final when ignorance and fear are overcome by proper observance of all laws pertaining to the creation of bones, flesh and blood.

Working knowingly with the Master Cleanser and Master Builder brings humanity closer to perfection of the human form.

Through eons past and on even into the present, man has been held and still remains in bondage of misery and suffering while witchcraft and quackery have run the gamut of the healing field of misinformation.

A group of simple and automatic laws of the master plan for creative living has given the sufferer his answers and release from his various forms of disease.

These laws pertaining to the construction and reconstruction of a more perfect body are unlimited within the universal plan for man.

Though we have seen and felt the action of these laws as they automatically create and recreate in our many phases of living we have discovered and used them knowingly, only in limited amounts.

To most of us these laws have been replaced with the laws of "Kill or Cure" with the many devastating action and reaction of destructive practices and miracle poisons.

These truths are self evident as we look into the history of our diseases and see our failures in our constant search for release. If these records are not enough then let him go on and on with his never ending aches and pains until his sufferings have finally created a desire for knowing these many truths.

When we finally become sick of being sick then we are ready to learn the truth and the truth shall set us free.

This diet will prove that no one needs to live with his diseases. Lifetime freedom from disease has become a reality.

At last a new field of healing has been brought to the world and for those who would listen and believe a new knowledge will set them free from the slavery of false conceptions.

At last the basic mystery of disease has been solved by the MASTER CLEANSER.

# THE MASTER CLEANSER

To be complete, a healing system must be able to cover the entire field of human experience – physically, mentally, and spiritually.

Any system which denies any part of this trinity fails in its attempt to heal to the same extent to which it denies any part or parts.

For the novice and the advanced student alike, cleansing is basic for the elimination of every kind of disease. The purpose of this book is to simplify the cause and the correction of all disorders, regardless of the name or names. As we eliminate and correct one disease we correct them all.

This program has been tested and approved for over twenty years in all sections of the continent as the most successful of any other diet of its type in the entire field. NOTHING can compare with its positive approach toward perfection in the healing field. Nothing can compare with its rapidity and completeness.

As the originator of this superior diet I most humbly and yet proudly offer this to you, confident that you too will receive the finest with its use.

*Most sincerely,*

Stanley A. Burroughs

# THE MASTER CLEANSER

## Preface

Disease, old age and death are the result of accumulated poisons and congestions throughout the entire body. These toxins become crystalized and hardened, settling around the joints, in the muscles and throughout the billions of cells all over the body.

It is believed that we have a perfectly healthy body and that something comes along to destroy it when actually the building material for the organs is inferior and thus the organs are inferior or diseased.

Lumps and growths of all kinds are formed all over the body as storage spots for unusable and accumulated waste products, especially in the lymphatic glands. These accumulations depress and deteriorate in varied degrees causing degeneration and decay. The liver, spleen, colon, stomach, heart and our other organs and glands come in for their share of accumulations thus impairing their natural action.

These growths and lumps appear to us as forms of fungi. Their spread and growth is dependent on the unusable waste material throughout the body. As the deterioration continues our growths increase in size to take care of the situation. Fungi absorb the poisons and try to take the inferior material from the organs. This is a part of Nature's plan to rid the body of our diseases. When we stop feeding these fungi and cleanse our system we stop their development and spread; then they dissolve or break up and pass from the body.

We spend a good share of our lives accumulating these diseases and we spend the rest of our lives attempting to get rid of them or die in the effort.

The incorrect understanding of the above truths have led many uncivilized and civilized nations to search for some magic "cure" in all kinds of charms, witchcraft and unlimited kinds of obnoxious poisons and drugs. In general they are worse than useless because they cannot possibly eliminate the cause of any disease. They can only add more misery and suffering and shorten one's life still further.

As we continue to search for more and more magic "cures" we become more and more involved with complicated varieties of diseases. A simple understanding and action has always proven to be the best to eliminate our negative actions and reactions.

Germs and viruses do not and cannot cause any of our diseases, so we have no need for finding various kinds of poisons to destroy them. In fact, man will never find a poison or group of poisons strong enough to destroy all the billions upon billions of these germs without destroying himself at the same time. These germs are our friends and if given a chance will break up and consume these large amounts of waste matter and assist us in eliminating them from the body. These germs and viruses exist only when we provide a breeding ground in which they can breed and multiply. They will never harm or live in a healthy body. They cannot live in that type of vibration. Do you think that if an insignificant microscopic microbe can appear and make you sick when you were well and strong that you have any possibility of getting strong enough to throw them off at any time thereafter? Do you think that any destructive poisons can make it possible for you to get well any faster?

All types of disease, regardless of their names, come within this understanding as only the one disease of toxemia.

Deficiencies do exist, primarily because of improper diet and improper assimilation. These deficiencies also produce toxins because of the deterioration of the cells so we still have only the one disease. Thus we can approach the correction of these diseases as only one disease and with one simple plan we can eliminate all of them. As we eliminate these disease producing toxins from our body we must also rebuild these deficiencies. Thus a cleansing diet must also include proper material for building as the waste matter is eliminated.

The lemonade diet has successfully proven its worth consistently in its eliminative and building ability. It may be used with complete safety for every known type of disease.

The lemon is the richest source of minerals and vitamins of any food or foods known to man and are available the year around. Thus the diet may be used successfully any month of the year. Its universal appeal and availability make it pleasant and easy to use.

The lemonade diet first proved itself in the healing of stomach ulcers over twenty years ago. Since that time thousands of sufferers have testified to complete healing in only ten days. This is only one of the many miracles from which the user will find benefit.

As a reducing diet it is superior in every way to any other system because it dissolves and eliminates all types of fatty tissues. Fat melts away at the rate of about two pounds a day without any harmful after effect.

All mucous diseases such as colds, 'flu, asthma, hay fever, sinus and bronchial troubles are rapidly dissolved and eliminated from the body leaving the user free from the varied allergies which cause difficult breathing and clogging of the sinus cavities. Allergies exist as a result of an accumulation of these toxins and vanish as we cleanse our body.

These mucous disorders are brought about by the eating or drinking of mucous forming foods. In other words if you have these diseases you ate them. As we stop feeding our children mucous forming foods we can eliminate their mucous and allergy diseases for the rest of their lives.

The types of disease which form calcium deposits in the joints, muscles, cells and glands are readily dissolved and removed from the body. Cholesterol deposits in the arteries and veins also respond to the magic cleansing power of the lemonade diet.

All skin disorders disappear as the rest

of the body is cleansed. Boils, abscesses, carbuncles, and adenoids all come under this category. These conditions are again Nature's effort to eliminate poisons quickly from the body.

All types of infections are the result of these vast accumulations of poisons being dissolved and burned or oxidized to produce further cleansing of the body. Therefore rapid elimination of the toxins relieve the need for infectious fevers of all kinds. Infections are not "caught" they are created by Nature to assist in burning our surplus wastes.

Humanity builds a strong healthy body from the correct foods or it builds a diseased body from the incorrect foods. When disease does appear the lemonade will prove its superior cleansing and building ability.

# THE MASTER CLEANSER

— or —

# THE LEMONADE DIET

## Purpose

To dissolve and eliminate toxins and congestions that have formed in any part of the body.

To cleanse the kidneys and the digestive system.

To purify the glands and cells throughout the entire body.

To eliminate all unusable waste and hardened material in the joints and muscles.

To relieve pressure and irritation in the nerves, arteries and blood vessels.

To build a healthy blood stream.

To keep youth and elasticity regardless of our years.

## WHEN TO USE IT

When sickness has developed; in all acute and chronic conditions.

When the digestive system needs a rest and a cleansing.

When overweight has become a problem.

To assist in better assimilation and building.

Three to four times a year for all above uses and will do wonders for less serious or mild conditions. The diet may be done more often for serious conditions. Longer periods – up to forty days – may be safely followed for real serious cases.

## HOW TO MAKE IT

Combine the juice of one-half lemon or whole small lime (approximately two tablespoonfuls) and two tablespoonfuls of sweetening to an eight-ounce glass of medium hot water. The sweetening MUST be used to properly balance the lemon and to achieve the desired results of cleansing and building.

The various forms of sweetening may consist of all kinds of unsulphured molasses (Grandma's, Barbados, Louisiana, or Blackstrap). The various forms of molasses are slightly laxative. The most perfectly balanced sweetener of all is pure maple syrup and is the most desirable in taste appeal. Many people who have trouble with the other types of sweeteners find the maple syrup as the perfect answer. It is only condensed and not refined. The pure sorghum is the next best sweetener as it too, has not been refined or altered or adulterated. It is very tasty and of good quality.

These various sweeteners may be interchanged from time to time as one desires the change of taste. However, there is one exception. For those who have diabetes the blackstrap molasses must be used as it gives the necessary minerals the body needs for making the needed insulin and to make other balances in the blood sugar. The diabetic should start with only one teaspoonful of the molasses for each glass and then gradually increase the amount daily until the full amount is taken (two tablespoonfuls).

Honey must not be used at any time. It is

manufactured from the nectar picked up from the flowers by the bees, predigested, vomited and stored for their future use with a preservative added. It is deficient in calcium and has many detrimental effects for the human being. Honey is strictly for the bees.

Liquifying the skin and pulp and drinking that with the lemonade assists in cleansing by acting as a further laxative. At the same time it helps to give tone and quality to the blood. It enables the blood to clot properly at the surface and to be free from clotting in the veins and arteries. This can assist in correcting many types of hemorrhages. It also gives additional taste appeal. Adding a dash of cayenne pepper to each glass of lemonade will give an additional lift and is a blood building material.

The cayenne also helps to break up mucous and stimulate increased elimination of the toxins.

Mint tea may be used occasionally during this diet as a pleasant change and further assist in the cleansing. Its chlorophyll helps as a purifier, neutralizing many mouth and body odors that are released during the cleansing period.

## HOW OFTEN TO USE IT

Take from six to twelve glasses of the lemonade daily during the waking period. As one gets hungry just have another glass of lemonade. NO OTHER FOOD SHOULD BE TAKEN DURING THE FULL PERIOD OF THE DIET. As this is a more complete balance of minerals and vitamins one does not suffer the pangs of hunger.

All solid food is turned into a liquid before it can be carried by the blood. The lemonade is already a food in liquid form.

For those who are overweight less molasses may be taken. For those underweight more molasses may be taken. For those who are underweight and worried about losing more weight, REMEMBER, the only things that you can possibly lose are mucus, waste and disease. Healthy tissue will not be eliminated. Many people who need to gain weight do so near the end of the diet.

Never vary the amount of lemon juice per glass. About six glasses of lemonade a day are enough for those wishing to reduce. Extra water may be taken as desired.

## FURTHER INFORMATION

In case of too frequent eliminations of the intestinal tract, less molasses may be used. In case of insufficient elimination, more molasses may be taken separately if desired.

As this is a cleansing diet the more you can assist Nature to eliminate these poisons the better. REMEMBER if you are upset it is because you are not having sufficient

dian quart) teaspoonfuls of sea salt. Do not use ordinary iodized salt. Drink the entire quart of salt and water first thing in the morning. The salt and water will not separate but will stay intact and quickly wash quite thoroughly the entire tract in about one hour. Several eliminations will likely occur. The salt water has the same specific gravity as the blood, hence the kidneys cannot pick up the water and the blood cannot pick up the salt. This may be taken as often as needed for proper washing of the entire digestive system. If the salt water does not work the first time try adding a little more or a little less salt until the proper balance is found; or possibly take extra water with or without salt. This often increases the activity. Remember, it can do no harm at any time. The colon needs a good washing but do it the natural way – the salt water way.

It is quite advisable to take the herb laxative tea at night to loosen, then the salt water each morning to wash it out. If for some reason the salt water can not be taken in the morning then the herb laxative tea must be taken night and morning.

Some people want to take pills or food supplements on the diet. This does not always produce the desired result. There are many reasons. As the lymphatic glands become clogged they are no longer able to assimilate and digest even the best of foods. As we cleanse our body and free our cells and glands of toxins that clog and paralize our assimilation we free our various activities to do their proper job. Note on page 29 that all the vitamins and minerals may be found in the lemonade and therefore do not need additional supply in most cases. Later as we consume a more complete variety of foods we find our source of vitamins and minerals complete in a form that is easily assimilated.

Our source of good food is steadily being enlarged as we educate the people. Search these sources and rely on them for your food.

The lemon is a loosening and cleansing agent with many important building factors. Its 49% potassium strengthens and energizes the heart, stimulates and builds the kidneys and adrenal glands; its oxygen builds vitality; its carbon acts as a motor stimulant; its hydrogen activates the sensory nervous system; its calcium strengthens and builds the lungs; its phosphorus knits the bones, stimulates and builds the brain for clearer thinking; its sodium encourages tissue building; its magnesium acts as a blood alkalizer; its iron builds the red corpuscles to rapidly correct all forms of anemia; its chlorine cleanses the blood plasma; its silicon aids the thyroid for deeper breathing.

The molasses, sorghum, or maple syrup is an eliminator and builder. It also contains the Woolsen loosening factor. The natural iron, copper, calcium, carbon and hydrogen help to build the blood to normal, and gives plenty of energy. It truly is a perfect combination for cleansing, eliminating, healing and building.

In the cleansing process, some people experience a tremendous stirring up; and, possibly feel worse for several days. It is not the lemonade which causes the trouble but what the lemonade stirs up in the system that causes our dizziness and other disturbances. Vomiting may occur under certain conditions; increased pain may be felt in the various joints of the body; even dizziness may develop on certain days. If weakness develops at any time, it is the result of poisons circulating through the blood stream, rather than a lack of food or vitamins. This diet gives a person all the vitamins, food and energy necessary for the full ten days or longer, in a liquid form.

Even though the lemon is an acid fruit it becomes alkaline as it is digested and assimilated. It is our finest aid toward the proper alkaline balance.

Alcoholics, smokers and other drug addicts will receive untold benefits from this diet. The chemical changes and the cleansing remove the craving and the many possible deficiencies. Thus the desire for these unnatural types of stimulants and depressants disappear. The usual cravings experienced and suffered in breaking away from drugs, alcohol and tobacco no longer present themselves during and after this diet.

It is truly a wonderful feeling to be free from slavery to these many habit-forming and devitalizing articles of modern living. Coffee, tea and the various cola drinks, as habit-forming beverages, also are readily conquered with the marvels of the lemonade diet.

## What to Do After Ten Days

*The 11th Day:* Drink as much orangeade (half orange juice – fresh – and half water –with or without the natural sweetening as mentioned on page 19) during the day as is desired. Some time during the afternoon, prepare a vegetable soup (no canned soups) with several kinds of vegetables, such as one or two kinds of legumes, potatoes, celery, carrots, green vegetable tops, onions, etc. Dehydrated vegetables or vegetable soup concentrates may be added for extra flavor. Okra or okra powder, chili, curry, cayenne (red) pepper, tomatoes, green peppers, and Zucchini squash may be added to good advantage. Brown rice also may be used but no meat. Have this soup for the evening meal using the broth mostly, although some of the vegetables may be eaten. Rye wafers may be eaten sparingly with the soup, but no bread or crackers.

*The 12th Day:* Drink the orangeade in the morning. At noon have some more soup; enough may be made the night before and put in the refrigerator. For the evening meal, eat whatever is desired in the form of vegetables, salads, or fruit. No meat, fish or eggs; no bread, pastries, tea, coffee or milk. Milk is highly mucous forming, and tends to develop toxins throughout the body. Milk, being a predigested food, has been known to cause various complications in the stomach and colon, such as cramps and convulsions. The calcium in the milk, being difficult to assimilate, may cause toxins in the form of rheumatic fever, arthritis, neuritis, and bursitis. The resulting lack of proper digestion and assimilation of the calcium allows it to go into the blood stream in a free form and is deposited in the tissues, cells and joints, and can cause intense pain and suffering.

*The 13th Day:* Normal eating may be resumed, but best health will be retained if the morning meal consists of our type of lemonade, fruit juice, or vegetable juice. For proper assimilation of the various forms of food, drink one or two glasses of lemonade one hour before each meal. At the end of each meal, take one or two Papaya tablets: and with your meal, sip a glass of warm water with two teaspoonfuls of pure Apple Cider Vinegar (Sterling brand or any good country variety) added. This helps to produce digestion, and eliminates fermentation and formation of gas. If, after the 13th day, eating causes distress or gas, it is suggested that the lemonade diet be continued for another three or four days until the system is ready for food.

## FOR BEST HEALTH

Follow the fruit, nut and vegetarian way of eating; it causes less congestion and chronic or acute disorders. Keep the body clean, inside and out.

NOTE: This diet is given merely as a suggestion; anyone who follows it does so voluntarily. Since each person, naturally, reacts differently, each individual should use his own judgement as to its use.

### Exercise

The importance of exercise cannot be

stressed too strongly. Since we have a body we must use it to its fullest. Walking is excellent the same as other types but best of all is stretching, bending and twisting. We do a great deal of this in our work if it is quite strenuous but this is not enough. Slant board exercise is also important. It is good to figure out a regular system of these exercises and do them daily.

## WATER FASTING

The subject of water fasting often presents itself. I am very much opposed to several days or weeks of water fasting. It is too dangerous and unnecessary to achieve the desired results.

Many people are already deficient as well as toxic. The longer they do without food the greater becomes the deficiency. The lemonade diet can more than match all the possible good obtained from fasting and at the same time help rebuild any possible deficiency.

Ordinarily with fasting it is necessary to take it easy by resting or staying in bed. On the contrary, with the lemonade diet there is no need to become a useless member of society and you may live an active, normal life. Many workers at hard labor have often found they are able to do more and harder work on the lemonade diet than on the normal diet.

After one has attained a clean, healthy body and then desires to fast for purely Spiritual reasons, then thirty or even forty days can cause no harm. First we must build our physical body to its highest form.

Friends and acquaintances may find this diet to be the answer to their aches, pains or other troubles. Even if there appears to be nothing wrong sometimes those who are "never sick" will feel so much better. Let your friends receive this benefit too.

## DROPSY

Dropsy is one of our most difficult and least understood of many diseases of toxemia. Varied attempts to correct this condition has met with little or no success. The main treatments can give only temporary relief and the final result, as these treatments fail to produce any change, is death from internal drowning.

To achieve fast relief and lasting correction one must completely understand the causes.

This unusual and simple approach to an ancient disease will achieve fast and lasting results. As in so many other diseases, dropsy is a vast accumulation of toxic waste. These toxins accumulate because our eliminative organs are unable to take care of them as fast as they enter or are formed in the body. As accumulations steadily increase they first appear to us in a liquid form. If they are not eliminated from our body they are automatically and gradually dehydrated or crystalized. They are then deposited in any and all of the available spaces throughout our cells, glands and organs. This continues until a saturation point is reached and then Nature reverses the action and slowly dissolves the crystalized and dehydrated material. This change makes a final effort to save the life from being snuffed out from complete stoppage of all glands and organs. Only in a liquid or semi-liquid form can we eliminate our toxins. Usually by this time our eliminative organs are over worked and clogged, our heart, liver and kidneys suffer the most, so they cannot carry off the liquid toxins. The body then steadily increases in size until it can no longer sustain life.

The correction for this fatal condition is simple, fast and effective. Just follow directions and the results will be most satisfactory.

## The Treatment

Start the patient off on the lemonade diet. Secure one hundred (100) pounds of coarse rock salt (may be bought at a feed store). Cover the bottom of the bath tub with about two inches of salt. Unclothe the patient and wrap them in a wet sheet. Lay the patient on the salt and add salt to about two inches above their body so that the entire body is surrounded with the salt. The room should be 80° or slightly higher so the patient does not get chilled. The tub may be warmed first with hot water before adding the salt. Let ALL the water out first before adding the salt.

Leave the patient in the salt for close to one hour. Be sure and give them several glasses of hot lemonade with the cayenne pepper.

Remove the patient from the salt and wrap them in a woolen blanket to keep them warm. Extra heat may be used if necessary. Repeat this treatment every other day or daily if not too weak from the rapid changes.

This may be repeated until all the swelling has gone down or the toxins are removed. The first application may not produce notable results but from then on a rapid change should be noted.

Be sure to keep them on the lemonade diet until a big change has taken place even if it continues for ten, twenty or thirty days. Color and Vita-Flex may be used also with tremendous increased action and elimination.

IMPORTANT – NOTE: The salt may be used over and over on the same patient but not on any other. *Each person must have their own salt.*

Bathing one or two times a day especially

during this diet is specifically necessary. We eliminate wastes through the breathing, the skin, the kidneys, the colon and from the sinus through the nose. The most wastes are eliminated by breathing, and next in their order the skin, the colon, the kidneys and depending on the individual from the sinus. Often we eliminate large quantities of wastes in the form of mucous as we develop our colds, 'flu, etc. One can see how important becomes our elimination by the skin. Even when in good condition it is important to bathe once or twice daily to remove these wastes from the surface of the skin thus allowing it to breathe properly. These baths will help to eliminate these obnoxious odors while we cleanse our body.

## MENU SUGGESTIONS

Due to the fact that our system goes through a cleansing process from twelve midnight until twelve noon and a building program from twelve noon to twelve midnight, anything eaten during these periods must conform to the natural processes.

*For Breakfast:* Fresh lemonade, other fresh fruitades or juices or various fresh vegetable juices with water added for better assimilation. Various herb teas are of great benefit. One of the finest of these for a quick and lasting lift is a combination of two parts of peppermint, one part each of spearmint and wintergreen leaf teas. It has a marvellous and bracing effect on the entire body. It gives such a clean feeling and is a wonderful tonic. As many cups or glasses may be taken as desired, but no solid food. Maple syrup, sorghum, or molasses may be added for extra taste if desired.

*Noon Lunch:* A small vegetable or fruit salad may be used to great advantage. Soup (homemade) or tomato juice, hot or cold, may be had with the vegetable salad. Coconut milk or almond milk may be taken with the fruit salad.

NOTE: Recipes for coconut and almond milk, and a number of dressings are to be found at the back of the book.

*Dinner:* Simple preparations for dinner can be had by starting with a vegetable soup then two or three vegetables steamed slightly. On other occasions special dishes such as vegetable stew, various types of brown rice dishes (curried rice, spanish rice, chop suey and rice), chili beans made with lima beans or red beans, or any recipe using lentils and garbonzas but no meat. Vegetarian cutlets and all prepared meat substitutes should be used very sparingly. Here is a simple suggestion for a dish.

Equal amounts of tomatoes, egg plant and okra with various spices added makes a very unusual dish.

All kinds of berries are good for lunch or dinner.

## COCONUT OR ALMOND MILK

6 tbsp. powdered coconut or almonds
3 cups water
¼ cup maple syrup
1 small banana
Liquify for 5 minutes.
¼ cup raw cashews may be added to make it creamy. Also a little cinnamon and nutmeg may be added for extra flavor.

## FRUIT SALAD DRESSING

½ cup water
½ cup maple syrup
4 tbsp. coconut – powdered or fine
2 tbsp. sesame or soya bean oil
½ cup raw cashews
1 slice fresh pineapple if possible.
Cinnamon and nutmeg if desired.
Liquify for 5 minutes.

## VEGETABLE SALAD DRESSING

½ cup olive oil or good cold pressed oil
½ cup pure apple cider vinegar
¼ cup maple syrup
1 large fresh tomato
1/5 tsp. cayenne pepper
1 tsp. powdered mustard
½ tsp. paprika
Dash of tumeric, chili powder, oregano and sage.
1 clove garlic
Juice of 1 lemon or lime and rind of a quarter of it.
Salt

Liquify for 5 minutes. Quarter cup of raw cashews may be added to make it creamy.

Mayonnaise Dressing — following the above recipe, leaving out the tomatoes and garlic.

## DRESSING FOR COLE SLAW

2 tbsp. raw cashews
¼ cup oil (cold pressed)
¼ tsp. powdered cloves
¼ tsp. ginger
¼ cup maple syrup (approx.)
⅛ cup apple cider vinegar
Salt
Juice of whole lemon
1 slice pineapple ¾ x 4″
¼ tsp. soy lecithin granules

Liquify for 5 minutes.
If a thinner dressing is desired add water.

Broken pieces of cashews will be found to be less expensive.

### Basic Recipe for Milk

6 tbsp. raw sesame
6 tbsp. raw cashews

In a liquifier two speed or more powerful grind the above dry and until fine. Fill liquified with water and mix.

This basic drink may be used for a large variety of drinks and frozen desserts. This may also be used to make a cream sauce for a large variety of steamed vegetables. It also can be used in soups, scalloped or creamed potatoes, creamed vegetables, etc. It is used just as you would use milk. The best thickener to use is brown rice flour.

### Basic Cream Sauce and Thickener

To the above after grinding and before adding water add 3 tbsp. brown rice flour, salt, 2 tbsp. cold pressed oil, then fill liquifier with water and run liquefier for a few minutes to combine. Pour this into the hot vegetables and stir rapidly while thickening.

## Basic Ice Freeze

6 tbsp. raw sesame
6 tbsp. raw cashews

Grind very fine as mentioned before. Then add ½ cup cold pressed oil, approximately ½ cup maple syrup or raw sugar.

Mix 2 tbsp. agar agar in 1 cup water and cook until completely dissolved and add to above. Then add any flavor desired such as fresh strawberries, raspberries, pineapple, etc.

To make simulated chocolate add 7 tbsp. carob.

To make a little more creamy add 2 tbsp. gum arabic (made from grapes).

For best results use an electric or hand freezer. If it is frozen in ice trays it will not have a smooth texture but will be sort of crystalized instead of creamy. One liquifier makes approximately 1½ quarts. Make as many liquifiers full as you need to fill your freezer. Have the liquid at least 1½ inches from the top of the freezer as it expands in freezing.

Always make the mixture a little sweeter than desired as some of the sweeting is lost in freezing.

*May this cleansing diet be a most glorious beginning to the very best in your work and play and the many hours of complete relaxed rest and undisturbed sleep.*

*May this bring to you many more disease-free years. Truly the* MASTER CLEANSER *can prove that Creative Living is a reality.*

*As this work proves its worth, further knowledge and experience will be desired. The finest in the healing field is Vita-Flex and Color. They, too, will prove there can be a more perfect correction for all disorders.*